The Winner's

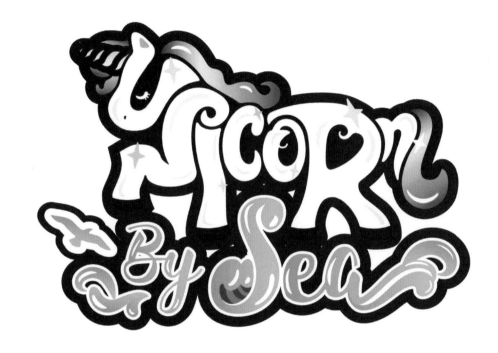

The Unicorn by Sea Chronicles

Michael Peace

Michael Peace

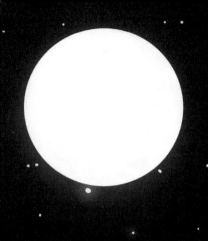

Hidden away in a town by the sea, a secret doorway exists with your imagination as the key. For when the moon is full and bright, a magical and sparkling world comes into sight. Down by the old fort on the edge of the beach, the world opens up and your dreams are in reach. Full of unicorns, mermaids, fairies and more, all of them wonderful, with hearts pure. So if you are willing to truly believe, these wonderful creatures a story will weave. They invite you to let your dreams run free into the magical world of Unicorn by Sea.

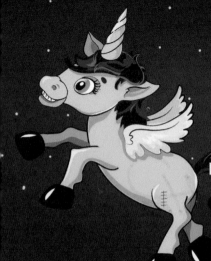

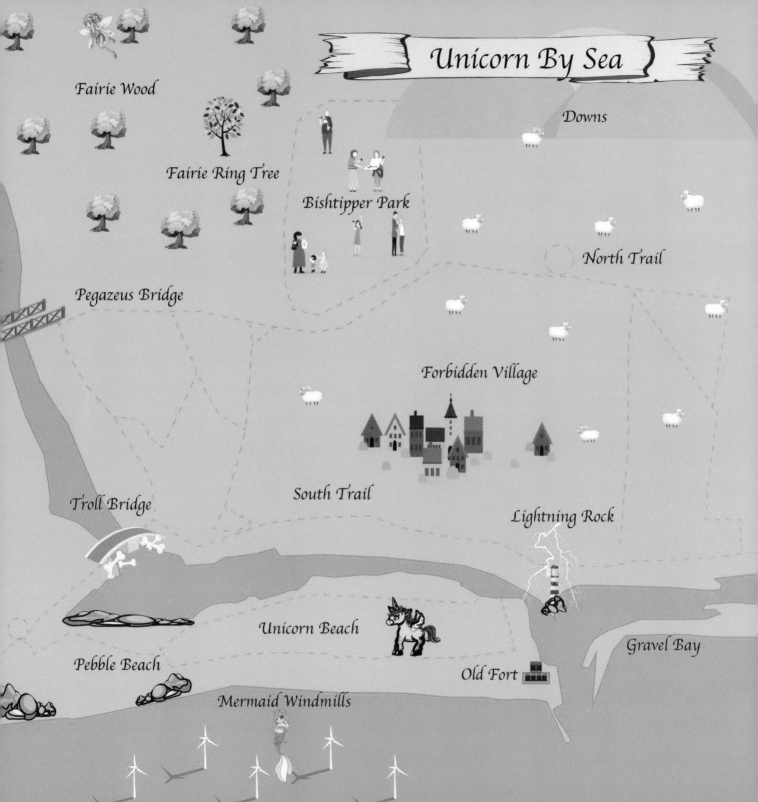

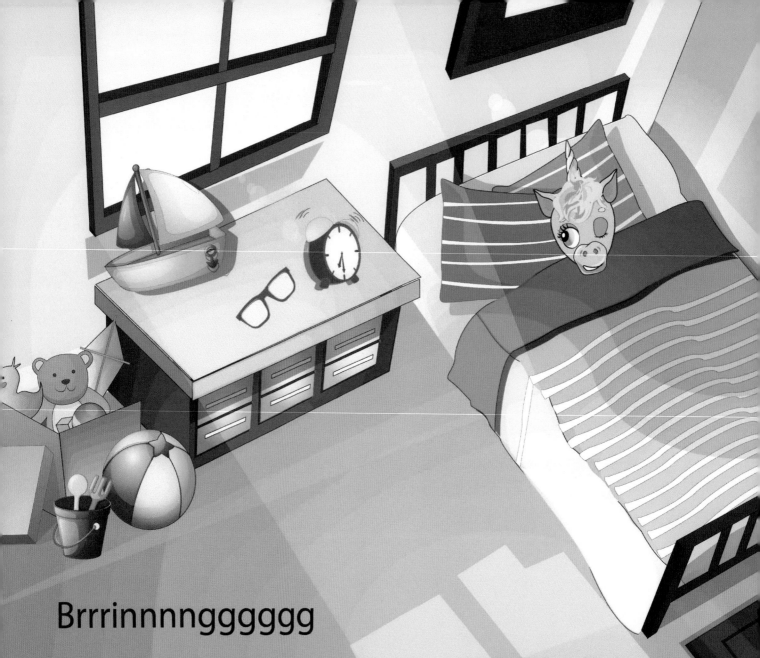

Brrrinnnngggggg

The alarm clock woke Sparky and he opened one eye and looked at his calendar.

Suddenly excited he shouted "It's the great race today and I'm taking part for the first time."

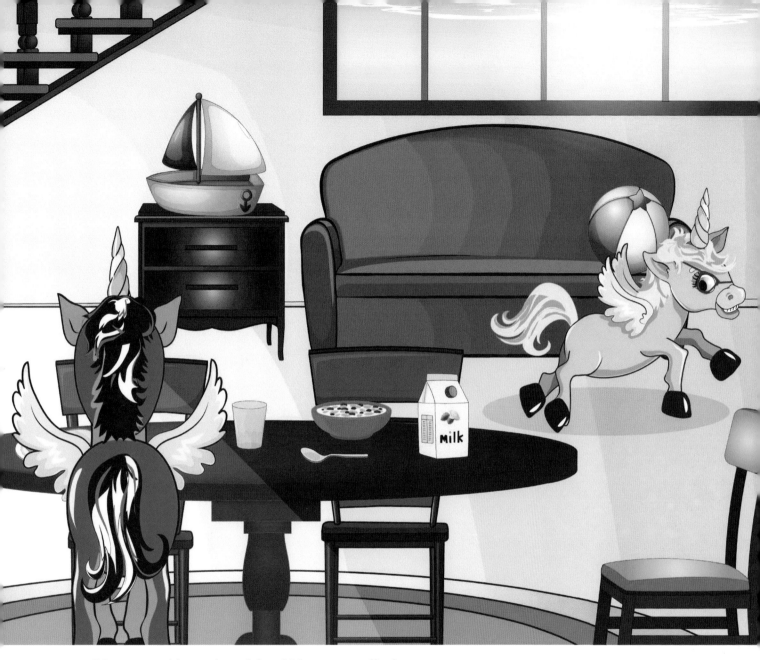

"Come and have breakfast" Mummy called.

"I'm too excited for breakfast Mummy, it's race day and anyway, I'm not hungry!"

"My friends are here" Sparky shouted and ran out of the door.

Sparky told his friends "I'm so excited for the race, I wasn't hungry and I couldn't eat breakfas

"I sometimes don't feel hungry either" said Rocky "but it's the most important meal of the da especially on race days and that's why I had an extra large breakfast."

Sparky laughed "Really? I think you'll be too full to run after all that food. Haha I'm going to beat you to the finish line."

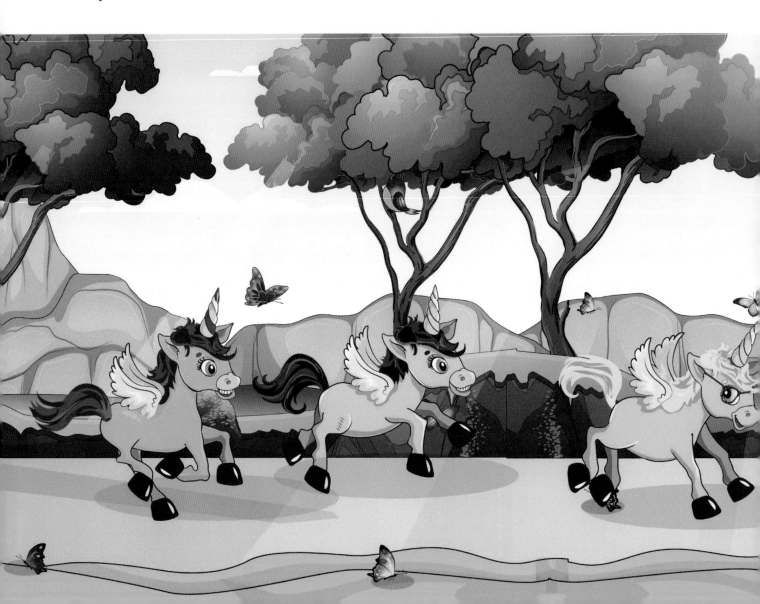

When they arrived at the beach, Sparky gasped "Wow look at all these unicorns, I need to run really fast at the start to get ahead, otherwise I may get trampled."

The unicorns all lined up and the race began.

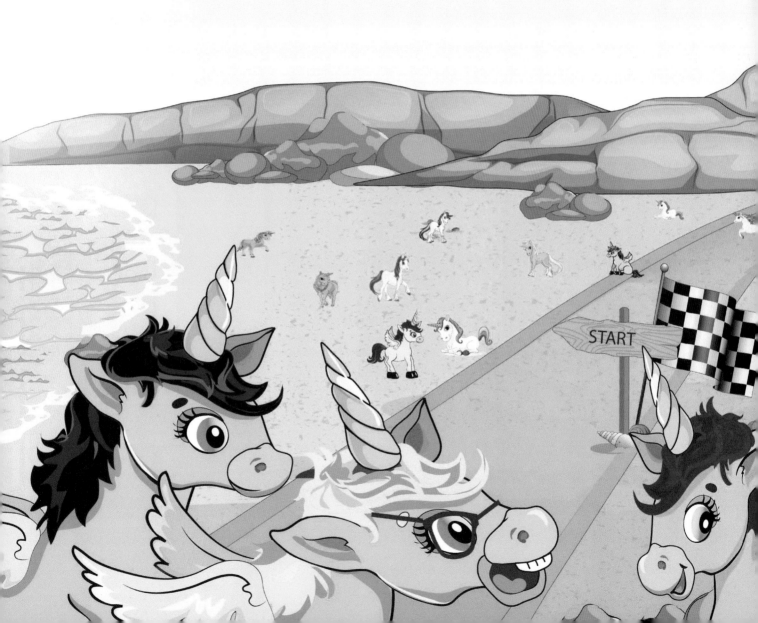

"Wow these rocks are hard to climb, it's really tiring."

"Keep going Sparky you're over half way" shouted Rocky in the distance.

But Sparky was starting to slow down...

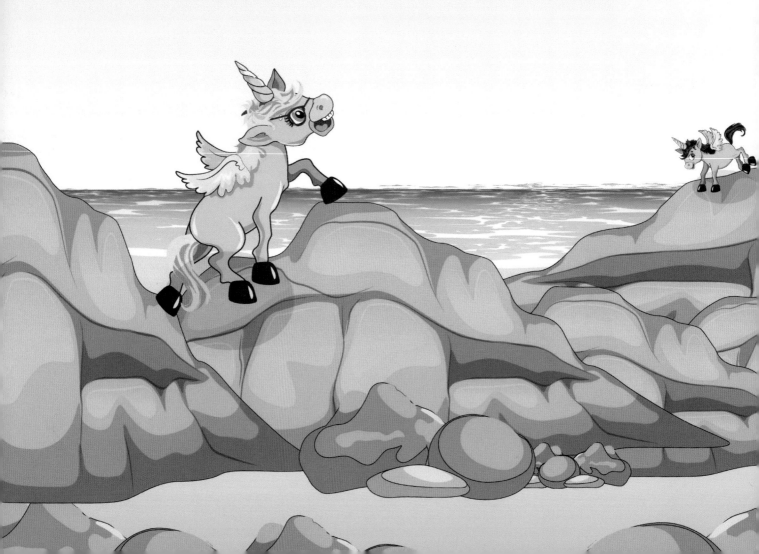

All the other unicorns had finished the race by now and poor Sparky had stopped.

"I'm too tired, I can't go any further, I've just got no energy."

Rocky looked down remembering Sparky had missed breakfast. "I'll come down and help you."

Rocky helped Sparky to get home.

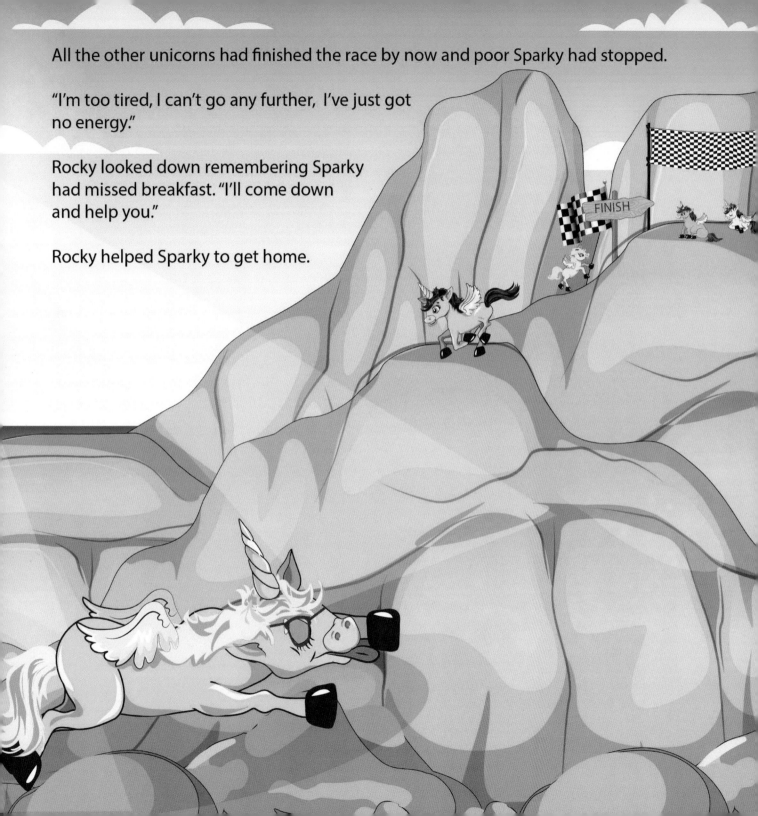

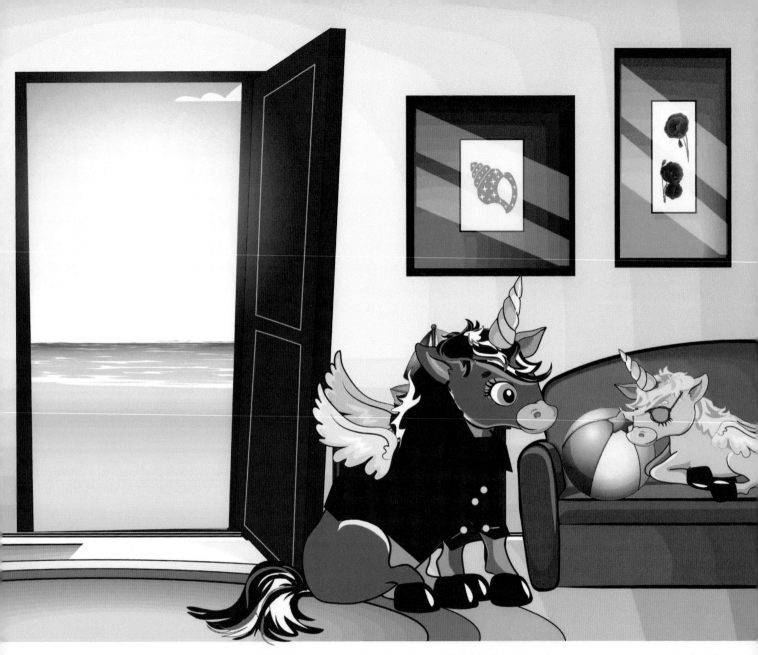

"How did the race go?" Mummy asked, "I couldn't finish the race! I started well and was near the front, but then when it became difficult I just ran out of energy."

"Oh dear, that's because you had no breakfast. I know just how to help, Daddy always has porridge before a race and he says it helps him run longer."

URGH PORRIDGE!

"I hate porridge, Nana tries to feed it to me all the time and it tastes horrible!"

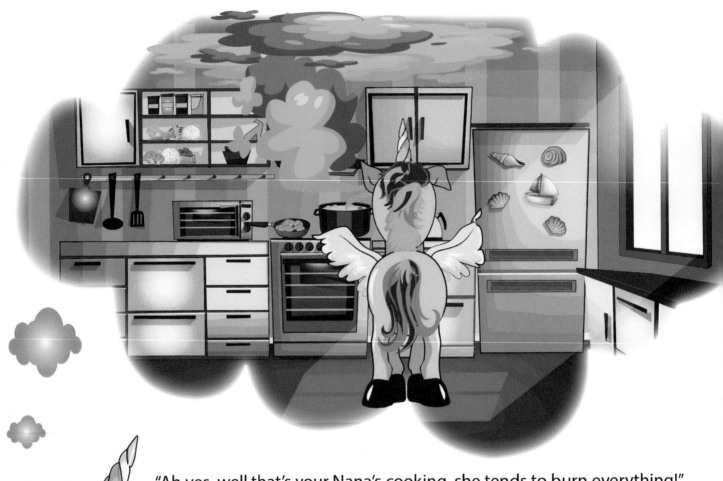

"Ah yes, well that's your Nana's cooking, she tends to burn everything!"

"If you overcook things, they do taste horrible."

"Your porridge should be light and fluffy and it tastes a lot nicer if you add some honey and fruit or berries to it."

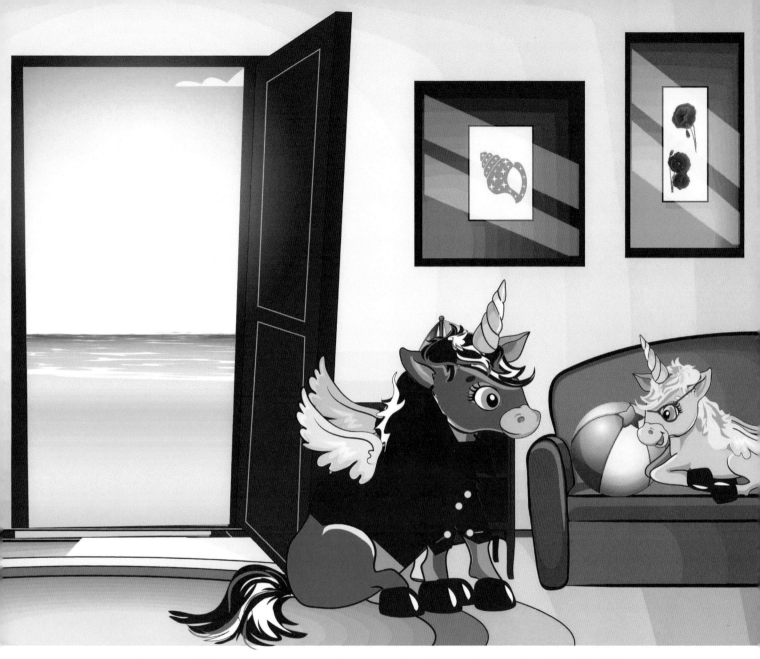

"Really? Could I try some porridge tonight then please, just like Daddy eats?"

"And Mummy" asked Sparky, "Yes?"

"Please don't tell Nana", "of course not" Mummy whispered smiling.

"Wow, this porridge is so yummy it tastes amazing" Sparky squealed with delight.

"It's like eating a completely different food to Nana's."

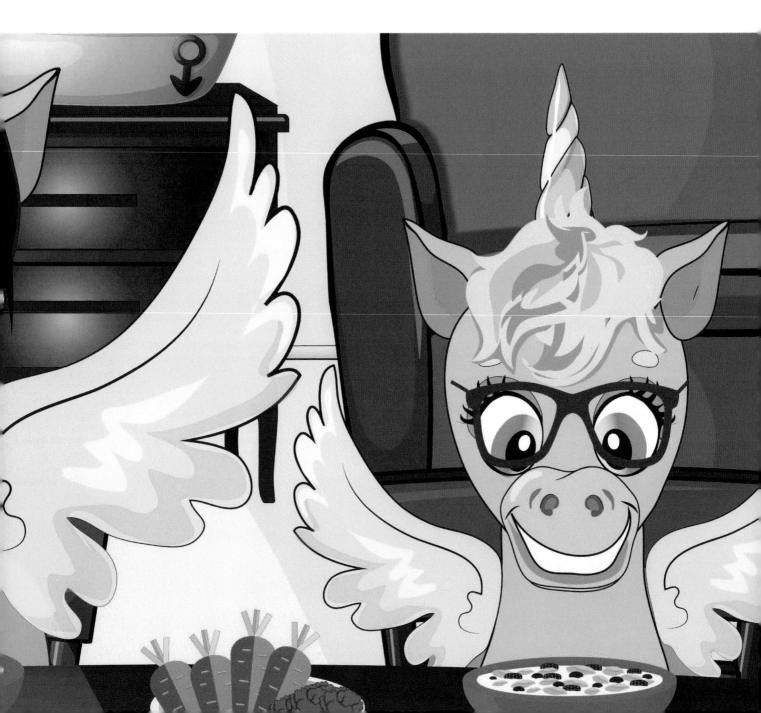

"Porridge is my favourite" said Daddy "I have it every day at breakfast with a smoothie, it helps build up my strength and energy."

"No wonder you couldn't finish the race, breakfast is the most important meal of the day. If you have porridge for breakfast tomorrow, I bet you will finish the race."

Sparky smiled "porridge is my favourite now too!"

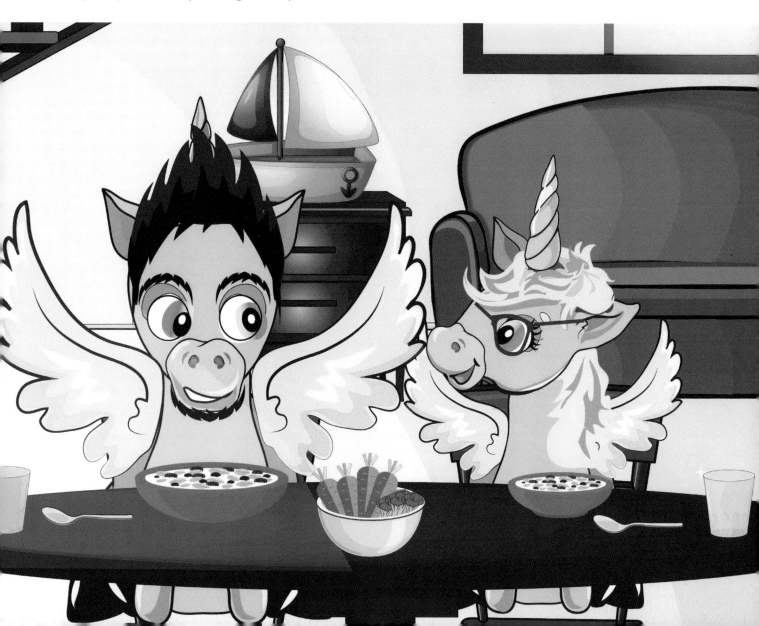

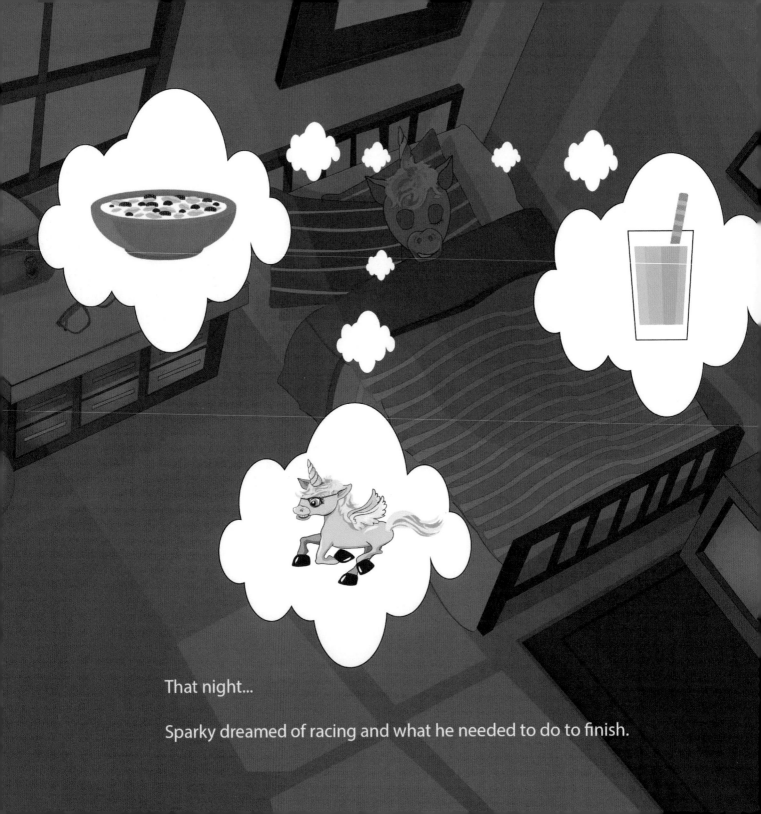

That night...

Sparky dreamed of racing and what he needed to do to finish.

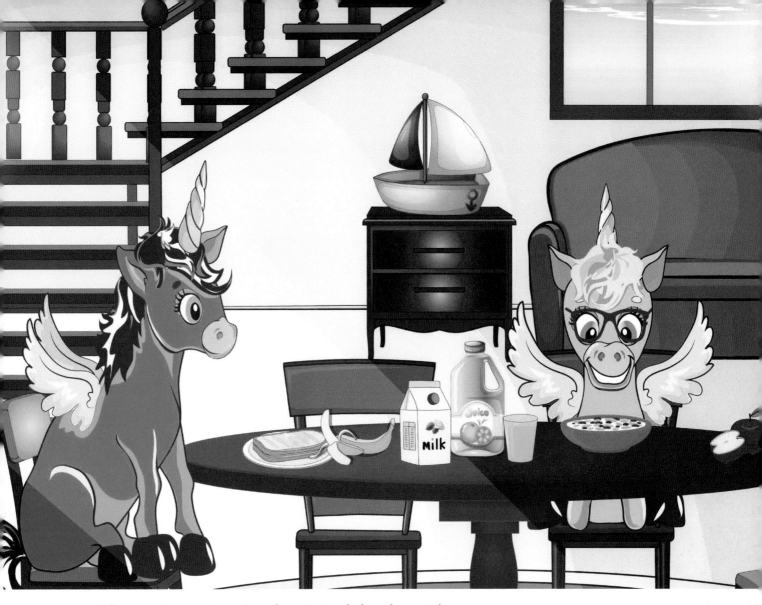

The next morning Sparky started the day with...

"Porridge with bananas and honey, a smoothie and some toast - Yummy! This is going to give me lots of energy."

"That's a breakfast for winners, I'm sure you're going to finish today's race."

"Thanks Mummy" answered Sparky "I believe that as well!"

"I'm so excited for today's race - I had an extra big breakfast" Sparky told his friends.

"I did as well - I had oats and bananas" said Rocky, "I had fruit salad and toast" said Auriana.

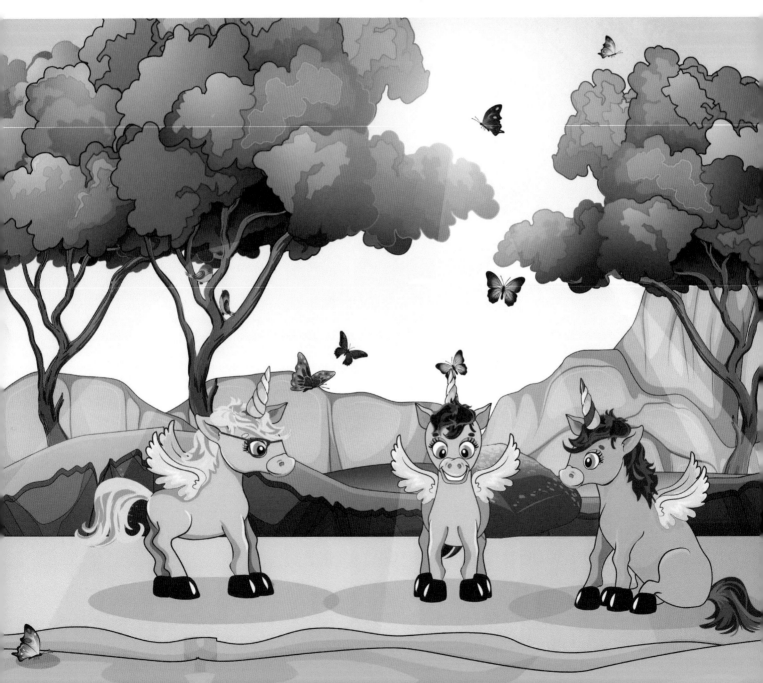

"I had all three" said Sparky "porridge with bananas and honey, toast and a smoothie."

"Wow" the others replied.

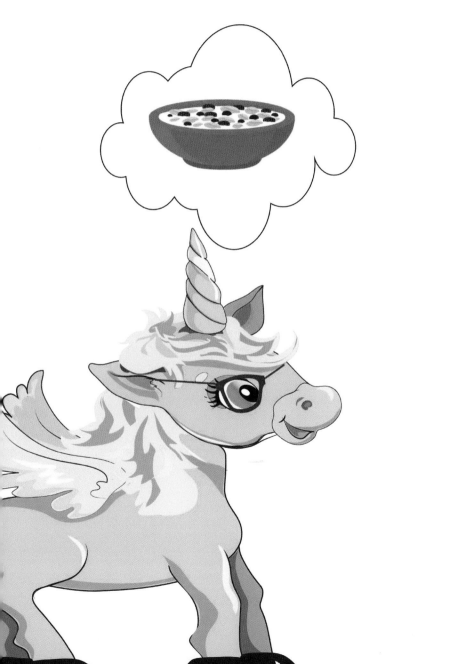

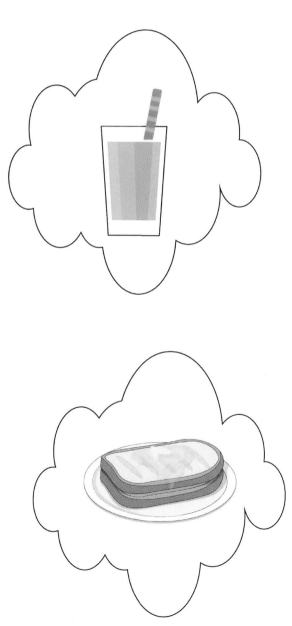

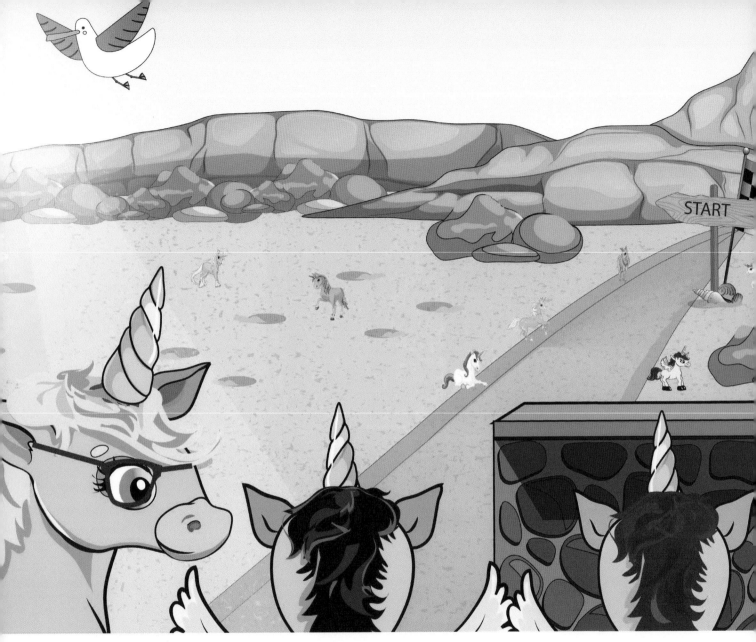

Down at the beach the unicorns were getting ready.

"Gosh - its another busy race." said Rocky.

"Hmm I definitely need to go fast at the start to get ahead of the crowd" whispered Sparky to himself and then the race started!

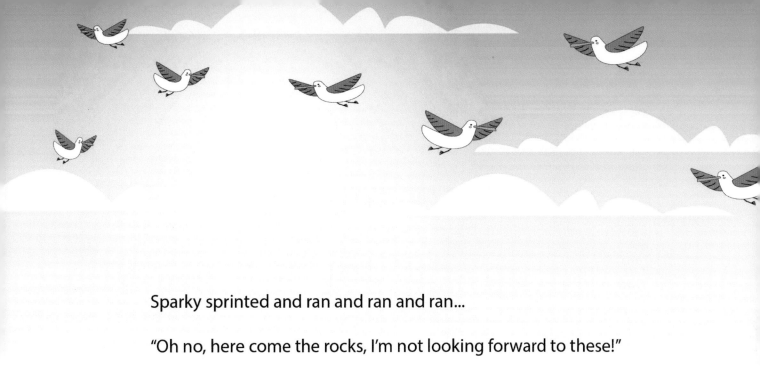

Sparky sprinted and ran and ran and ran...

"Oh no, here come the rocks, I'm not looking forward to these!"

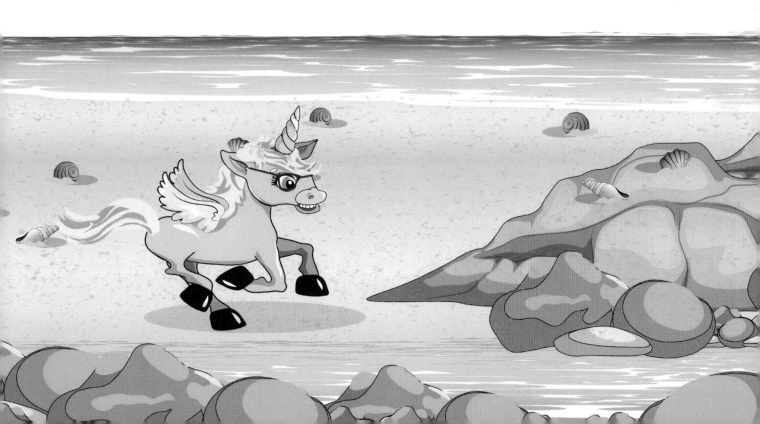

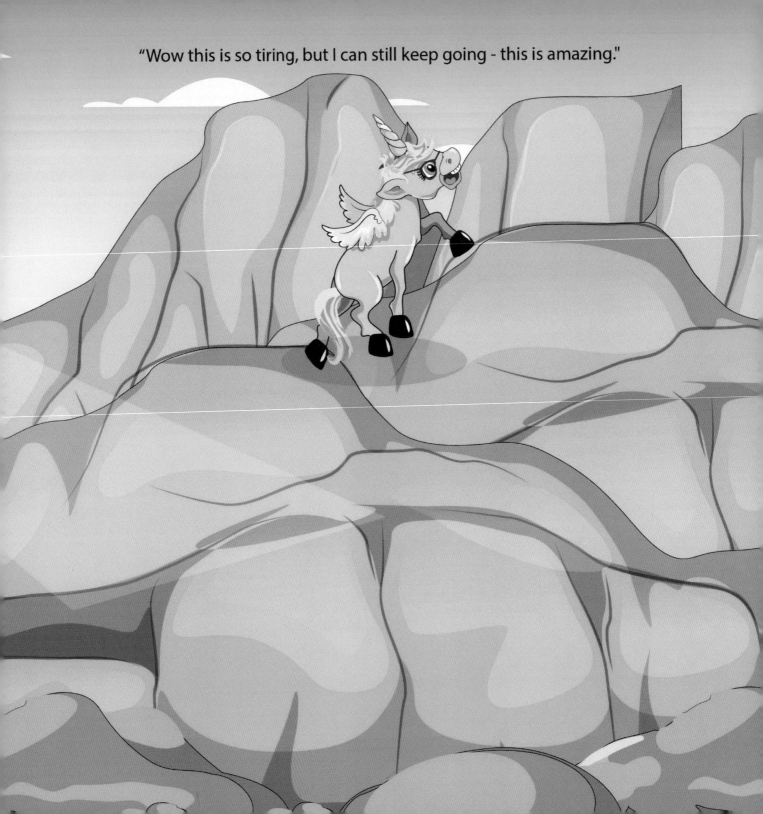

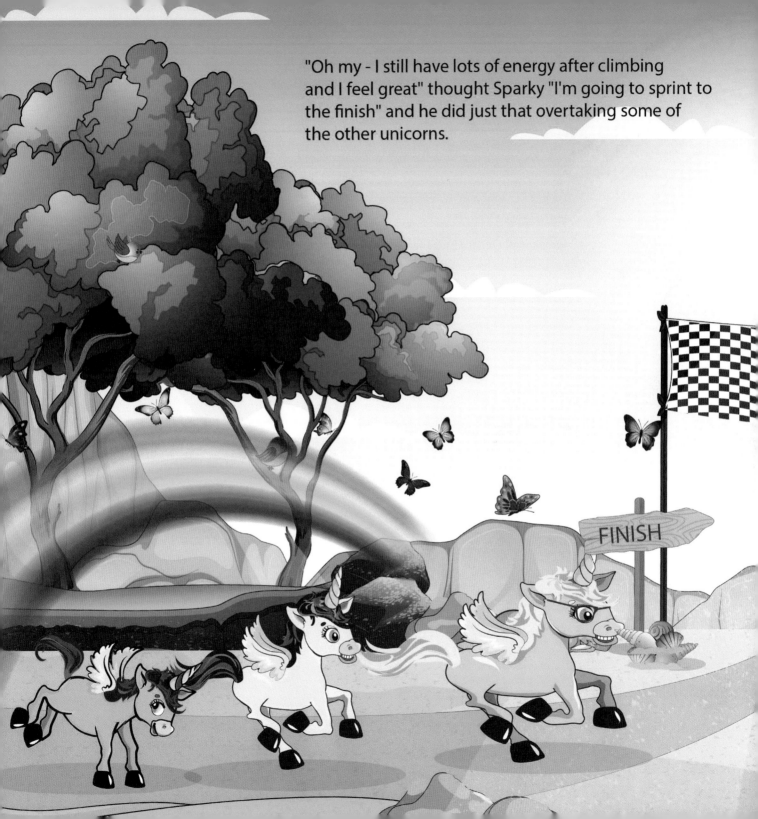

"Oh my - I still have lots of energy after climbing and I feel great" thought Sparky "I'm going to sprint to the finish" and he did just that overtaking some of the other unicorns.

"Wow, that was a fantastic race" said Rocky, "well sprinted at the end, you're going to get a star for that."

Sparky beamed with happiness "I knew I was a good runner, but I didn't realise how important breakfast was for energy. It sure is the most important meal of the day."

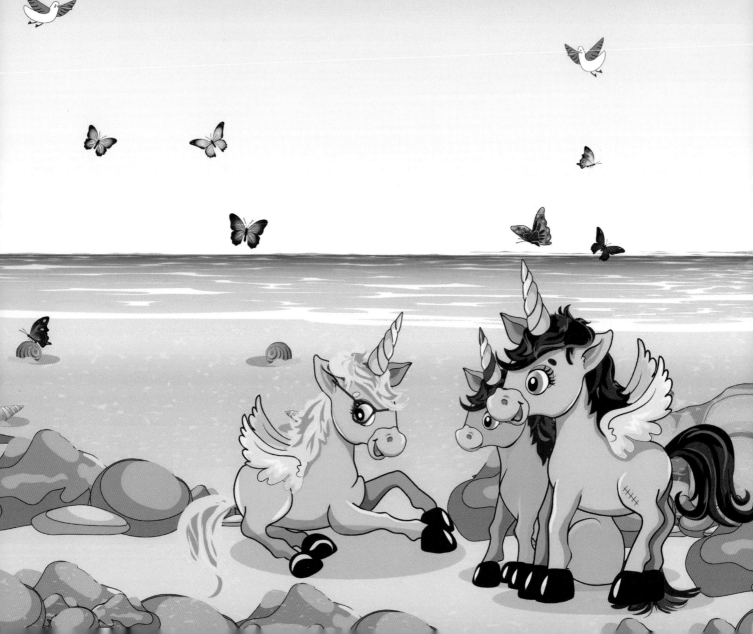

It was time for the judges to announce the winners.

"In third place we have Auriana, in second place is Sparky and the winner of the Great Unicorn Race is Rocky!"

Sparky's friends clapped with delight, "second place that's great - well done Sparky!"

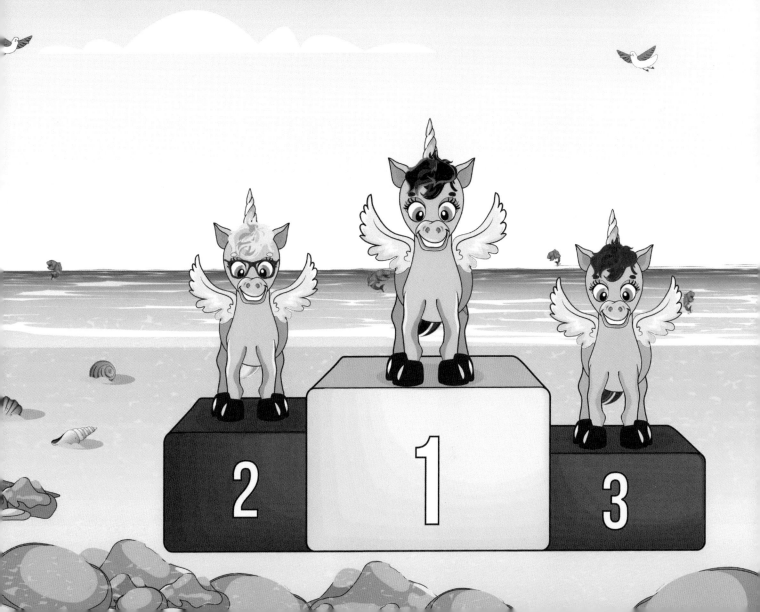

"Breakfast is the winner's secret!" shouted Sparky showing off his unicorn winner's star" and everyone cheered!

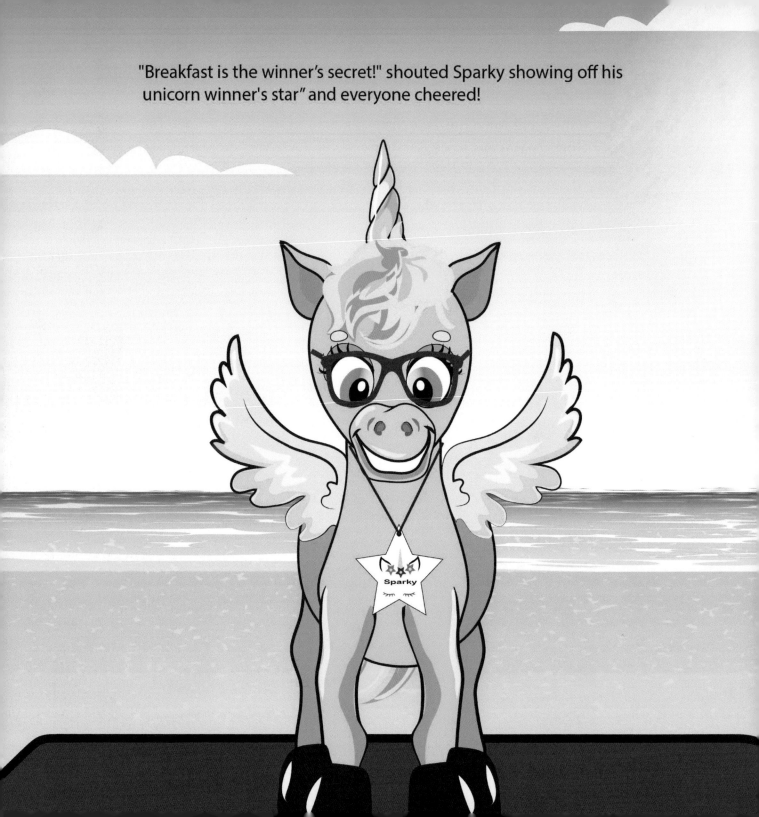

The Great Unicorn Race. Help Sparky find a winning route!

START

FINISH

Profile - Sparky

Favourite Juice: Green Boost

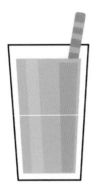

1/2 Lemon

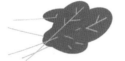

1 Cup Spinach

1 Kiwi Fruit

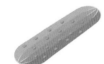

1/2 Cucumber

1 Cup Broccoli

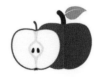

2 Apples

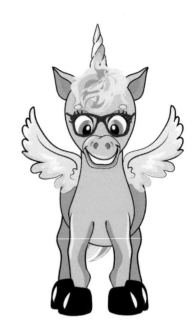

Favourite Food   Favourite Snack

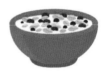

Porridge   Bananas

Favourite Hobby

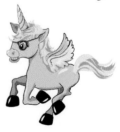

Running

Available from:
www.unicornbysea.com

The Unicorn by Sea Chronicles

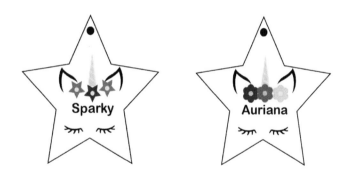

Personalised Unicorn Stars

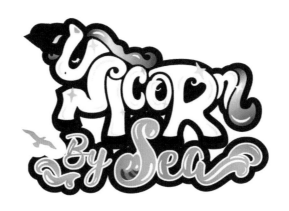

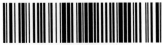

44043036R00019

Printed in Poland
by Amazon Fulfillment
Poland Sp. z o.o., Wrocław